YOUR KNOWLEDGE HAS VALUE

- We will publish your bachelor's and master's thesis, essays and papers

- Your own eBook and book -
  sold worldwide in all relevant shops

- Earn money with each sale

Upload your text at www.GRIN.com
and publish for free

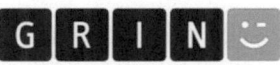

Bibliographic information published by the German National Library:

The German National Library lists this publication in the National Bibliography; detailed bibliographic data are available on the Internet at http://dnb.dnb.de .

This book is copyright material and must not be copied, reproduced, transferred, distributed, leased, licensed or publicly performed or used in any way except as specifically permitted in writing by the publishers, as allowed under the terms and conditions under which it was purchased or as strictly permitted by applicable copyright law. Any unauthorized distribution or use of this text may be a direct infringement of the author s and publisher s rights and those responsible may be liable in law accordingly.

Imprint:

Copyright © 2006 GRIN Verlag
Print and binding: Books on Demand GmbH, Norderstedt Germany
ISBN: 9783668940543

This book at GRIN:

https://www.grin.com/document/475181

Timothy John Whittard

Interprofessional Module 2. Who benefits from inter-professional working?

GRIN Verlag

GRIN - Your knowledge has value

Since its foundation in 1998, GRIN has specialized in publishing academic texts by students, college teachers and other academics as e-book and printed book. The website www.grin.com is an ideal platform for presenting term papers, final papers, scientific essays, dissertations and specialist books.

Visit us on the internet:

http://www.grin.com/

http://www.facebook.com/grincom

http://www.twitter.com/grin_com

Interprofessional Module 2

What was your group goal?

The following goal was explored within the interprofessional group:

> Who benefits from interprofessional working?

The learning outcomes selected by the group were:

a.) Explore ways to promote user participation within the provision of services.

b.) Promote and establish effective communication and working in teams to achieve interprofessional collaboration.

Group statements:

1.) Working collaboratively with other professionals in a multi-disciplinary team improves patient care.

2.) Communication barriers inhibit successful interprofessional working.

3.) Professionals should work together towards a common goal.

4.) Cohesiveness is not always evident within teams, and can take time to develop.

5.) Power can influence and manipulate people; and can be misused.

6.) Conflict of opinion can be healthy within a group, as this can highlight different views.

7.) Rules will only work if they are accepted and respected within the team.

8.) Interprofessional education is about learning about the roles of other professionals.

9.) Mutual support and respect helps team cohesion.

10.) Everybody is a potential service user.

11.) Effective collaborative working can require compromise.

12.) The patient is central to the delivery of care.

13.) Poor interprofessional collaboration can lead to confusion and an impersonal experience for the patient.

14.) There is a need to improve standards of interprofessional working.

Select four statements from the list compiled by the group, and explain why they are relevant to your own learning about interprofessional collaboration.

The four statements I have selected are numbered 1, 2, 13 and 14 (in the above list).

    The first statement here is undoubtedly relevant to my own learning about interprofessional collaboration, as I have found that it is frequently reported that successful collaboration between healthcare professionals leads to improvements in the provision of care for patients. This message was reinforced throughout the interprofessional conference, during many of the lectures and seminars; and is supported by Kaas et al (2000) who report that the quality of care delivered to patients is "highly dependent" on the collaborative efforts between healthcare professionals. Furthermore, it is reported by the NHS (2003) that good interprofessional working creates improvements in "the experience and outcome of care for patients".

Lax and Galvin (2002) emphasise that poor communication presents a barrier to interprofessional collaboration, which inhibits its success; a view that supports and reinforces the second statement. This became apparent following the conference, when the interprofessional group encountered difficulty with the online aspect of the work. This presented a challenge, as it was difficult to acquire input from all of the group members, possibly due to the need for internet access to communicate with one another. DiMeglio et al (2005) report that good communication between professionals is conducive to collaboration and teamwork; a view supported by Daly (2004) who argues that a high standard of communication "is the linchpin of successful collaboration".

The significance of the thirteenth statement is highlighted by Roberts and Priest (1997), who state that inadequate or poor interprofessional collaboration can lead to "confusion and misunderstandings", and detracts from the making of progress. This was evident during the group work sessions at the interprofessional conference, when at times, members of the group became unsure about and confused by the tasks that had been set, and what was expected of them; inevitably this cost the group valuable time. Furthermore, Rushmer (2005) reports that such confusion, and the blurring of professional boundaries can "lead to resentment and distrust". Carlick and Price (2006) state that good collaboration between professionals can lead to improvements in the 'patient experience'; therefore, conversely, one may argue that poor collaboration could detract from the experience of our patients.

Headrick et al (1998) and Daly (2004) both highlight the relevance of the fourteenth statement, reporting that there is a need to improve standards of interprofessional collaboration; in addition, Sloper (2004) states that this need is widely recognised. This is relevant to my own learning because it validates my participation in interprofessional education as a student healthcare professional. Furthermore, Barr (2006) emphasises the need to learn from past mistakes and errors, which may have been avoided, and were contributed to through "ineffective interprofessional working".

<u>Word count – 432 words.</u>

What have you learned during this module?

Attending the interprofessional conference has clearly been beneficial; I feel that this has provided me with an experience, which has enriched my understanding of the processes involved in interprofessional collaboration, and has also raised my awareness of the inherent difficulties or barriers that may arise. Furthermore, the conference repeatedly stressed the need for professionals to keep the patient at the heart of the collaborative process, and also promoted the involvement of the patient at every possible juncture; this is echoed by the first learning outcome selected by the group, and is supported by Toop (1998) who describes a "partnership" between the patient and the professionals, emphasising the importance of "patient participation" throughout the decision making processes. Headrick et al (1998) agree, stating that the needs of the patient must be the "explicit focus" of collaborative efforts, in order to achieve the best possible outcome.

The need for good communication skills when working in an interprofessional situation was highlighted both during and after the conference; the second learning outcome chosen by the group reiterates this notion. At times during the interprofessional group work sessions of the conference, and whilst completing the online aspect of the conference work, it became clear that communication difficulties were creating uncertainty and confusion (Roberts and Priest, 1997), which in turn, was causing the group to lose direction (Hill and Ingala, 2001). This also highlights the need for good leadership, as it is suggested by Amos and Herrick (2005) that an effective leader is vital in order to "plan, coordinate, and monitor" the activities of the group, whilst also "inspiring team collaboration". This may have helped to maintain the direction of the group and may have helped to prevent or reduce the "breakdown in team function" (Madce and Khair, 2000). In addition to this, the NHS (2003) explains that good team leadership is "more likely to lead to sustained changes in service improvement".

Major (2002) highlights that "group cohesion" can take time to develop, this became clear at the conference; the interprofessional group did not function well initially, and time was required in order for a sense of 'team' to form. However, once the team had established itself, I feel that the group members were able to work well together, collaboratively, in pursuit of achieving the outlined goals. This demonstrated how professionals from different disciplines are able to work alongside one another, towards a common goal, for the benefit of the patient (Headrick et al, 1998).

Yuen et al (2006) state that interprofessional learning creates a "significant positive improvement" in the attitudes of the participants "towards learning and working with students from other professions". The conference provided me with the opportunity to learn from other professionals and students of different disciplines, and also fostered an environment that allowed the diverse experiences and knowledge of the participants to be shared. Mandy et al (2004) suggest that the conference facilitated the "mixing of professional groups" and encouraged "interprofessional discussion"; adding that this can contribute to an improved understanding of the roles of other professionals. This reinforces the need to value and respect the differing knowledge bases and "unique expertise that each member brings to the team" (Houldin et al, 2004).

The learning I have acquired from the conference can only be beneficial, and I feel that the knowledge I have gained here will be highly advantageous when working collaboratively in the future. Despite this, Kenny (2002b) reports that the term 'interprofessional working' continues to be "a poorly understood term in clinical practice"; therefore, one may assume that there is a need to share or cascade the insight gained into working collaboratively from the conference with fellow professionals in practice.

Word count – 610 words.

Pick an article and relate it to one statement.

The article I have chosen is:

> Mandy, A., Milton, C. and Mandy, P. (2004) Professional stereotyping and interprofessional education. *Learning in Health and Social Care* 3(3) 154–170.

The statement I have chosen is numbered 8 (in the above list).

In this article the authors discuss the impact of professional stereotyping on the success of interprofessional collaboration and education. The article reports that there is a well-documented history of "interprofessional rivalry, tribalism and stereotypes" within the field of healthcare; furthermore, the authors investigate the stereotypes held by student healthcare professionals of differing professional groups, "before and after a semester of interprofessional education". Their results suggest that the stereotypical views and opinions held by the students, towards the other professional groups were reinforced following the interprofessional education programme. Despite this, the authors do not deny the potential benefits of interprofessional education, however they do propose that the timing of the delivery of such interprofessional education to student healthcare professionals is, perhaps "critical", if the reinforcement of professional stereotypes is to be minimised.

I feel that is relevant to my own learning, as I have encountered and observed the negative effects of professional stereotyping and rivalry, both in practice and at the conference; this is important as it is reported by Cox (2003) that conflict arising through preconceived ideas and professional stereotyping has a "negative impact on team performance effectiveness". At the conference I feel that this was especially demonstrated during the time allocated for coffee breaks and socialising, when a visible proportion of students appeared to be segregated into groups according to their professions. Within each discipline there appeared to be much keen discussion about the factors, which separated them from the other professions, as opposed to discussion about their similarities (Headrick et al, 1998). Roberts and Priest (1997) suggest that this behaviour may have been exhibited due to feelings of "fear and suspicion" regarding the other professionals; adding that this can be "divisive" and can create a "them and us" situation (Major, 2002).

The group statement I have selected highlights the need for professionals to possess an awareness and knowledge of the roles of other disciplines, and is implicit of a need to overcome stereotypes and rivalries in interprofessional collaborative situations (Daly, 2004). Fineberg et al (2004) support this view, reporting that the barriers to effective collaboration, which are posed by stereotyping and negative interprofessional attitudes "need to be replaced by familiarity and understanding of other disciplines". This suggests that interprofessional learning may facilitate the growth of an understanding of the roles of other disciplines, which in turn, may lead to positive or constructive changes in stereotypical views regarding other professionals (Sloper, 2004).

According to Pollard et al (2004) stereotypes exist from the "outset of a professional programme"; and furthermore, Fineberg et al (2004) state that it is imperative to attempt to tackle issues of interprofessional stereotyping "early in interprofessional education". However, the authors of the article I have selected suggest that there is also a need to allow students to develop "a sound professional identity" prior to the initiation of interprofessional education; they propose that the "role insecurity" and "lack of professional identity", which is often experienced by newly enrolled student healthcare professionals can potentially lead to "inflexible role boundaries and a reluctance towards role sharing". Roberts and Priest (1997) support this argument, reporting that if interprofessional education is delivered at too early a juncture, then the territorial boundaries between disciplines may be fortified by a fear of the differences in experience and knowledge bases between those disciplines. This is important, as it is suggested by Toop (1998) that such an experience may "blur" professional boundaries, and furthermore Headrick et al (1998) add that this "diluted professional identity" presents a barrier to both interprofessional collaboration and interprofessional education.

The increasing drive and interest in interprofessional collaboration between healthcare professionals may be "perceived" to be "eroding and diluting" the boundaries between disciplines (Kenny, 2002a); the authors of the article I have chosen state that therefore, there may be advantages in delaying the commencement of such interprofessional education programmes for student healthcare professionals until "after a period of clinical exposure", suggesting that this may allow the students to develop a feeling or sense of belonging to their chosen profession, and that in turn, the students may become more open and receptive to collaborative education. Conversely, Daly (2004) argues that any such segregation in the education of healthcare professionals cultivates "professional arrogance".

Interprofessional education initiatives should have a placed emphasis on the exploration of the "similarities and differences" between professionals with the intention of highlighting the "complementary contributions" of different disciplines and also fostering mutual respect for both "colleagues and their expertise" (Fineberg et al, 2004). Kenny (2002a) supports this notion, declaring that the emphasis of collaborative education should be placed on learning "from and about" other professionals, adding that this may lead to more effective collaboration "across professional boundaries", to better meet the needs of the patient.

I feel that my understanding of the causes and impact of professional stereotyping on the success of interprofessional collaboration and education has been contributed to enormously through both attending the conference and reading this article. This has reiterated that professional stereotypes are not conducive to interprofessional collaboration, and that there is a need to educate professionals to avoid the use of such stereotypes in order to achieve successful interprofessional working. According to Sloper (2004) interprofessional education can potentially serve to raise an awareness of barriers to interprofessional collaboration and issues such as professional stereotyping. Furthermore, Lax and Galvin (2002) state that it is important for healthcare professionals to possess the ability to recognise and acknowledge barriers to interprofessional working, such as stereotypes, if those professionals are to contribute to the minimisation and prevention of such barriers; this carries clear implications for all healthcare professionals working collaboratively within a multidisciplinary team.

Word count – 936 words.

How could you take this into practice in the future?

In my opinion, it is unquestionable that this module has allowed me to gain much useful knowledge and a colourful insight into working collaboratively with professionals of other disciplines; I feel that the conference also delivered a rich opportunity to witness first-hand some of the potential facilitators and barriers to interprofessional working, which may be encountered in practice. The challenge is now to find appropriate ways of bringing this learning into a clinical setting for the benefit of patient care.

Madge and Khair (2000) report that the "success or failure" of interprofessional collaborative efforts are largely reliant on the "enthusiasm and dedication of each individual member"; implying a need for all healthcare professionals to make a conscious effort to promote and facilitate effective interprofessional working. Eilertsen et al (2004) and Carelick and Price (2006) both support this view, suggesting that individual healthcare professionals are themselves responsible for the efficiency and effectiveness of collaborative working. Therefore, I believe that by attempting to improve my own interprofessional skills and practices, other improvements in interprofessional working may perpetuate.

The need to improve standards of collaboration between healthcare professionals is emphasised by Kenny (2002b) who reports that instances of poor interprofessional collaboration in the past have caused the "fragmentation of care, patient dissatisfaction and poor outcomes"; furthermore, it must not be overlooked that some extreme examples of poor collaboration in the past have also lead to the avoidable death of patients (Hader, 2005). Bianchi-Sand (2003) adds that interprofessional working practices need to improve in order to "safeguard against preventable errors" such as these. This is also implicit of a need to possess effective communication skills, a view supported by Rolls et al (2002) who report that poor communication between professionals has been "consistently identified as inhibiting interprofessional working"; this became evident at times during the conference and also when working online, therefore I will endeavour to enhance and improve my interprofessional communication skills and will also attempt to be more mindful of differences in professional language between disciplines, with the intention of reducing the occurrence of interprofessional misunderstandings and confusion (Roberts and Priest, 1997 and Rushmer, 2005).

In addition to this, Daly (2004) illuminates the need for good "written" communication and "quality record-keeping" amongst healthcare professionals; this need has also been highlighted at times during my clinical placements, where the inaccurate recording of important information has lead to errors and complications in the provision of patient care. Therefore, I feel that it is imperative that all significant information relating to our patients is recorded accurately, and shared appropriately between the relevant members of the multidisciplinary team; furthermore, Rushmer (2005) suggests that this can help to prevent and reduce the duplication or omission of work, and Amos and Herrick (2005) add that this can consequently lower costs, increase efficiency and also increase the provision of quality care. I will therefore make a sustained effort to use this knowledge in order to improve my clinical practice.

This assignment has also highlighted that improvements in the standard of communication may help to limit the potential causal of damage to collaborative processes by barriers between healthcare professionals, which are posed by the adoption of interprofessional stereotypes and stereotypical attitudes (Mandy et al, 2004); this reiterates the importance of avoiding the use of interprofessional stereotypes. Furthermore, Daly (2004) suggests that interprofessional stereotyping promotes and encourages interprofessional rivalry, and consequently facilitates the development of interprofessional "power struggles"; and therefore, leading to the presentation of yet another barrier to the success of collaborative working (Banerjee, 2006). Significantly, it is also noted by Mandy et al (2004) that "negative attitudes" and the use of stereotypes create undesirable tension and "contribute to work dissatisfaction and poor communication"; therefore, I feel that as a student healthcare professional it is vital to have an awareness of the dangers of interprofessional stereotypes, and I will also attempt to avoid the application of such stereotypes in practice.

By working collaboratively at the conference with student healthcare professionals of other disciplines, I was able to learn that each individual team member and profession has a valid and worthwhile contribution to make, which demands both respect and consideration. Fagin and Garelick (2004) emphasise the importance of this, suggesting that all members of an interprofessional team are mutually interdependent, adding that no single team member can operate or perform "independently" of their fellow team members. This stresses the need for mutual respect between professionals; Houldin et al (2004) acknowledge that such respect "may take time to emerge", however they also report that a lack of mutual respect between professionals has the potential to present an "insurmountable barrier to effective collaboration". Lax and Galvin (2002) concur, again emphasising the need for professionals to possess "mutual awareness and recognition" of the "valuable skills and experiences" of the professionals of other disciplines within an interprofessional team; they add that this may however require a "conscious effort" on the part of the individual. As a student healthcare professional, I feel that this carries significant implications for clinical practice; and therefore, in my future practice I will attempt to foster a collaborative working attitude, which both values and respects the "unique contribution" of each discipline involved, with the intention of optimising the "various skills" possessed within and across the team (Madge and Khair, 2000).

I feel that this assignment has provided me with a fruitful opportunity to expand and improve my understanding of the facilitators and barriers to good interprofessional working; and furthermore, I feel that this module has successfully enabled me to broaden my own "knowledge and perspectives" as a future healthcare professional (Eilertsen et al, 2004). It is reported by both Roberts and Priest (1997) and Headrick et al (1998) that the increased demand on professionals to work collaboratively is driven by the challenge to meet the increasingly complex needs of patients. Furthermore, Eilertsen et al (2004) emphasise that good interprofessional working is advantageous not only to the patient, but also to healthcare professional themselves. However, it is also important to note that the needs of the patient must remain the "explicit focus" of interprofessional collaboration (Headrick et al, 1998), if the successful delivery of 'holistic care" is to be achieved (Kenny, 2002b).

Word count – 1030 words.

Reference List

Amos, M. and Herrick, C. (2005) The Impact of Team Building on Communication and Job Satisfaction of Nursing Staff. *Journal for Nurses in Staff Development* 21(1) 10-16.

Banerjee, S. (2006) G98 ADHD: Collaboration Between Paediatricians and CAMHS. Does it Work? *Archives of Disease in Childhood* 91(1) 39.

Barr, O. (2006) Interprofessional Working in Health and Social Care - Professional Perspectives. *Nursing Standard* 21(12) 31.

Bianchi-Sand, S. (2003) It Takes a Team to Prevent Errors: Experts call for a team approach to safety. *American Journal of Nursing* 103(12) 89-90.

Carlick, A. and Price, M. (2006) Improving the fundamental aspects of patient care. *Nursing Standard* 21(1) 35-38.

Cox, K. (2003) The Effects of Intrapersonal, Intragroup, and Intergroup Conflict on Team Performance Effectiveness and Work Satisfaction. *Nursing Administration Quarterly* 27(2) 153–163.

Daly, G. (2004) Understanding the barriers to multiprofessional collaboration. *Nursing Times* 100(9) 78-79.

DiMeglio, K., Padula, C., Piatek, C., Korber, S., Barrett, A., Ducharme, M., Lucas, S., Piermont, N., Joyal, E., DeNicola, V. and Corry, K. (2005) Group Cohesion and Nurse Satisfaction: Examination of a Team-Building Approach. *Journal of Nursing Administration* 35(3) 110–120.

Eilertsen, M., Reinfjell, T. and Vik, T. (2004) Value of professional collaboration in the care of children with cancer and their families. *European Journal of Cancer Care* 13(4) 349–355.

Fagin, L. and Garelick, A. (2004) The doctor–nurse relationship. *Advances in Psychiatric Treatment* (10) 277-286.

Fineberg, I., Wenger, N. and Forrow, L. (2004) Interdisciplinary Education: Evaluation of a Palliative Care Training Intervention for Pre-professionals. *Academic Medicine* 79(8) 769-776.

Hader, R. (2005) Collaboration paves the way for better care. *Nursing Management* 36(1) 4.

Headrick, L., Wilcock, P. and Batalden, P. (1998) Continuing medical education: Interprofessional working and continuing medical education. *British Medical Journal* 316(7133) 771-774.

Hill, K. and Ingala, J. (2001) Build a dream team. *Nursing Management* 32(9) 37-38.

Houldin, A., Naylor, M. and Haller, D. (2004) Physician-Nurse Collaboration in Research in the 21st Century. *Journal of Clinical Oncology* 22(5) 774-776.

Kaas, M., Dehn, D., Dahl, D., Frank, K., Markley, J. and Hebert, P. (2000) A View of Prescriptive Practice Collaboration: Perspectives of Psychiatric-Mental Health Clinical Nurse Specialists and Psychiatrists. *Archives of Psychiatric Nursing* 14(5) 222-234.

Kenny, G. (2002a) Children's nursing and interprofessional collaboration: challenges and opportunities. *Journal of Clinical Nursing* 11(3) 306-312.

Kenny, G. (2002b) Interprofessional working: opportunities and challenges. *Nursing Standard* 17(6) 33-35.

Lax, W. and Galvin, K. (2002) Reflections on a community action research project: interprofessional issues and methodological problems. *Journal of Clinical Nursing* 11(3) 376-386.

Madge, S. and Khair, K. (2000) Multidisciplinary Teams in the United Kingdom: Problems and Solutions. *Journal of Pediatric Nursing* 15(2) 131-134.

Major, S. (2002) Dysfunctional teams: a health and resource warning. *Nursing Management* 9(2) 25-28.

Mandy, A., Milton, C. and Mandy, P. (2004) Professional stereotyping and interprofessional education. *Learning in Health and Social Care* 3(3) 154–170.

NHS (2003) *Teamworking for improvement: Planning for spread and sustainability* – [online]. Available from:
http://www.modern.nhs.uk/researchintopractice/14993/15038/5th%20(Teamworking).pdf [Accessed 17th October 2005].

Pollard, K., Miers, M. and Gilchrist, M. (2004) Collaborative learning for collaborative working? Initial findings from a longitudinal study of health and social care students. *Health and Social Care in the Community* 12(4) 346–358.

Roberts, P. and Priest, H. (1997) Achieving interprofessional working in mental health. *Nursing Standard* 2(2) 39-41.

Rolls, L., Davis, E. and Coupland, K. (2002) Improving serious mental illness through interprofessional education. *Journal of Psychiatric and Mental Health Nursing* 9(3) 317–324.

Rushmer, R. (2005) Blurred boundaries damage inter-professional working. *Nurse Researcher* 12(3) 74-85.

Sloper, P. (2004) Facilitators and barriers for co-ordinated multi-agency services. *Child: Care, Health and Development* 30(6) 571.

Toop, L. (1998) Primary care: core values: Patient centred primary care. *British Medical Journal* 316(7148) 1882-1883.

Yuen, S., Taylor, D., Heller, D., Hunt, L. and Emond, A. (2006) G208 Evaluation Of A New Undergraduate Interprofessional Learning Paediatric Prescribing Workshop. *Archives of Disease in Childhood* 91(1) 75.

YOUR KNOWLEDGE HAS VALUE

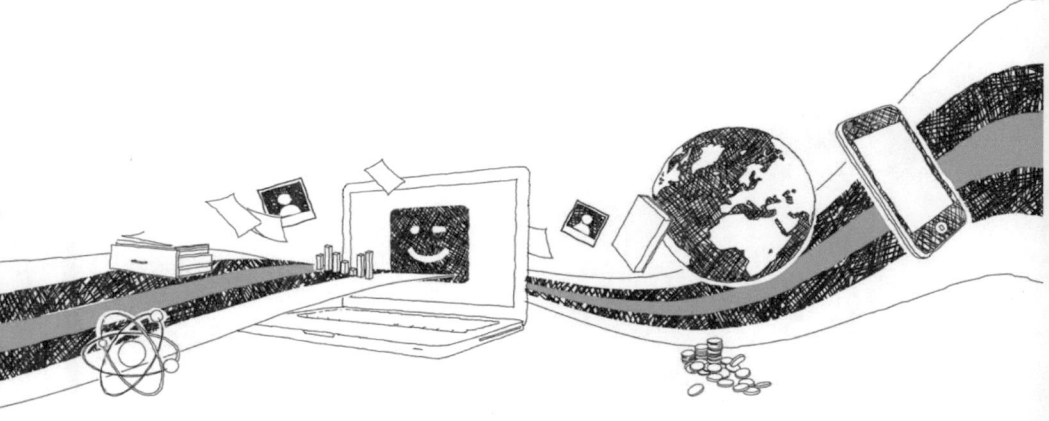

- We will publish your bachelor's and master's thesis, essays and papers

- Your own eBook and book - sold worldwide in all relevant shops

- Earn money with each sale

Upload your text at www.GRIN.com
and publish for free

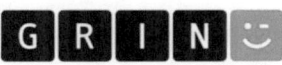